T0120273

Sexercise

Published in the United States by Cleis Press, an imprint of Start Midnight,
LLC, 221 River Street, Ninth Floor, Hoboken, New Jersey 07030.

Printed in the United States

10 9 8 7 6 5 4 3 2 1

Trade paper ISBN: 978-1-62778-321-7

E-book ISBN: 978-1-62778-534-1

Sexercise

F*ck Yourself Fit and Burn While You Bang

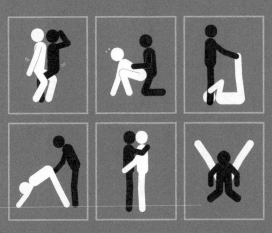

Wilma Fingerfit

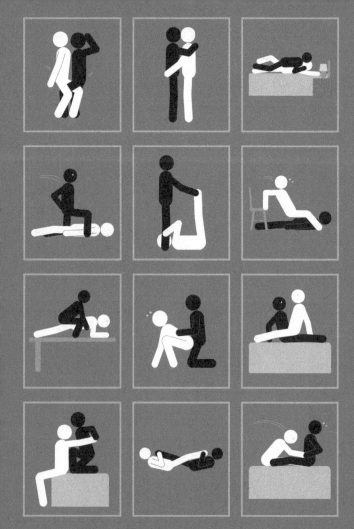

Contents

Introduction

Sexercise is a throbbing body of knowledge that will turn you into an elite sexual athlete in no time. First, work up a carnal appetite with some down and dirty warm-ups. Then find your rhythm with the beginner positions to get those juices flowing. Feeling the heat? Stay with the sweat and feel the sweet burn of some advanced bedroom acrobatics that will have you wailing like a hot-and-bothered banshee. And before you roll over and spoon the night away, don't forget that climactic cool-down. It's a wet and wild workout worth repeating again, and again, and again.

It's always advisable to speak to a health practitioner before starting a new exercise regimen. When it comes to sexercise, expect fanny flutters and wang wobbles from the get-go. Don't forget: consent is required and protection is perfection. You wouldn't go to the gym without wearing your sneakers, so come prepared and be prepared to come.

What the F*ck is Sexercise?

Sexercise helps you make the most of your bedroom antics, allowing you to transform your tired no-pants dance routine and up the acrobatic ante. These are downright dirty workouts that pump some serious love muscle—you'll definitely need a shower afterwards. Sweat your pants off, go balls to the wall, and take a trip to pound town that will leave you bulging all over.

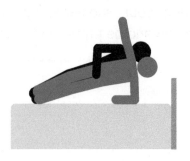

Equipment List

- A sturdy bed (or wherever else you like to do the dirty)

- Suitable sexercise apparel (e.g. lacy thong, leather chaps, nipple tassels)

- Toys to keep things interesting

- Your preferred method of contraception (stay safe, people!)

- All the lube you can handle

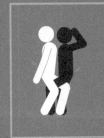
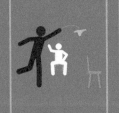
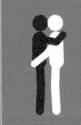
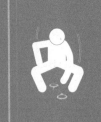
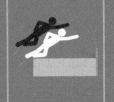
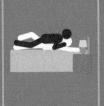
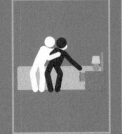
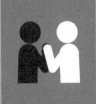
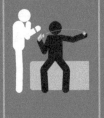

Warm-Ups

Whether you're *Fifty Shades of Grey* or fifty shades of greying, a few nifty stretches are the best way to prepare for a visit to bonksville. Before you get wild, get warmed up. Make sure your love muscles are locked and loaded and your nether regions are ready for the main event.

The Dry Hump

Don't panic, you're going to get laid. But before you're completely in the buff, take some time to practice your moves and find the perfect rhythm. Pick a body part and start grinding up against your partner—think ankle, elbow, left nipple . . . You'll work up a sweat and get other juices flowing too.

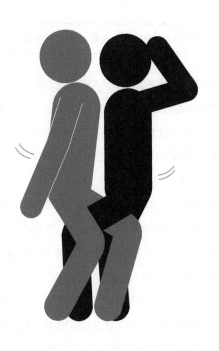

The Strip Teaser

Getting naked with your significant (or not-so-significant) other is a sure-fire way to get sex started. Avoid painful zipper incidents by slowly removing each item of clothing. Start with your own and then move onto your partner's if they're struggling. Wave it around in the air like you just don't care before tossing it, hammer-throw-style, across the room. Too easy? Take your throwing skills to the next level by aiming for specific targets; one point for a designated floor-drobe pile, two points for the chair, and five points for the laundry basket.

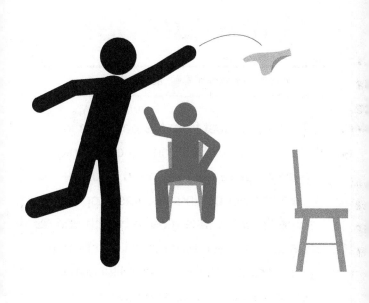

The Locked-Lips Limber

DIFFICULTY RATING: 🌶️🌶️ BURN RATING: 🔥

To get the most from the positions in this book and experience serious hanky-panky, you're going to need Popeye-worthy biceps and lithe lips. Apply some lip balm, take a deep breath and engage in some fervent tonsil tennis with your partner. While you kiss like crazy, embrace each other and stretch your arms as far around as you can. Don't forget to cop a feel if you desire it.

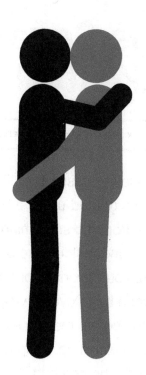

The Squat It Like It's Hot

DIFFICULTY RATING: 🍆🍆 BURN RATING: 🔥🔥🔥

Showcase your ass-ets while getting
your glutes geared up for a hump fest.
Practice dropping something sexually
essential on the floor (like a condom,
handcuffs, your favorite vibrator or a tube
of lube), then bend over, giving your lover
an eyeful, before moving into a squat
position to pick it up. Drop and repeat
till your thighs and butt are burning.

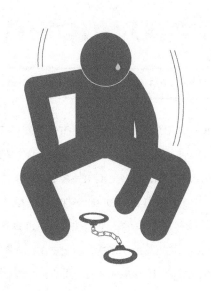

The Throwdown

Sooner or later, things are going to get physical. For your body and your furniture, it's a good idea to practice launching each other full-throttle onto the bed. Take it in turns to toss your partner into position, ensuring there's always a crashmat of duvets and pillows in place to protect them. Mastered this move? Try catapulting yourselves in unison.

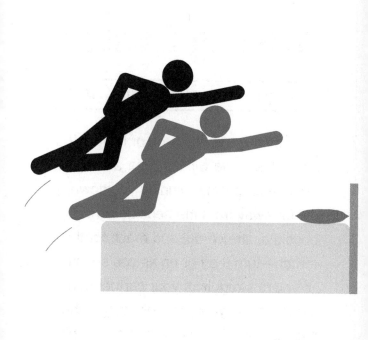

The Big Switch

Whether you're lights-on or lights-off lovers, this move will test your arm span. With your partner pinning you down as far away from the bedside light as possible, stretch out and reach for the switch—turn it off or on as you see fit. If you're struggling, your partner can reach across your face, giving you the chance to get intimate with their armpit.

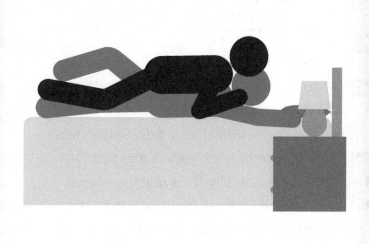

The Lubricator

There's nothing worse than a dry, chafey boning session: lubrication maketh sex. While it would be lovely if nature always stepped up with the goods, sometimes you have to take matters into your own hands. Literally. This reach-and-grab stretch for the lube tube in that little drawer by the side of your bed, while maintaining mouth-to-mouth kissing contact, should make sure you're nice and slippery at a moment's notice.

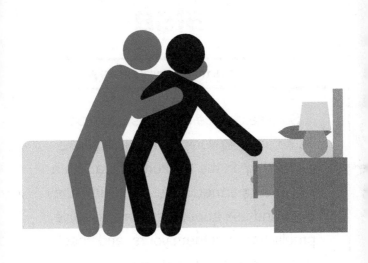

The Safe-Sex Salsa

DIFFICULTY RATING: ❘ BURN RATING: ❘

Safe sex is ace sex! This warm-up
is so easy, anyone can do it. If you're
embarking on the horizontal hula with a
brand-new partner, stare deeply into their
eyes and ask about their contraceptive
proclivities. Tell them yours, and check
everyone is all aboard for the next bit.
Blink a little to avoid straining your
eyes. Right, let's get to it then . . .

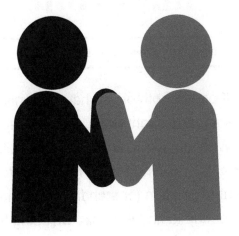

The Condom-nundrum

DIFFICULTY RATING: 👐 BURN RATING: 🔥

If one or both of you have a penis, someone might need to sheath up. When in doubt, shroud your spout! Practice moving from a horizontal to a seated position (or standing if you have to get up to find the box), whipping the condom out of the wrapper in record time and getting your little general dressed for battle. Ask your partner to time you so you can improve your performance for the next round.

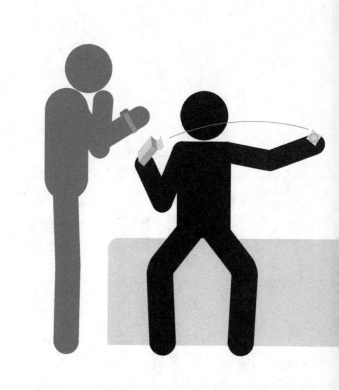

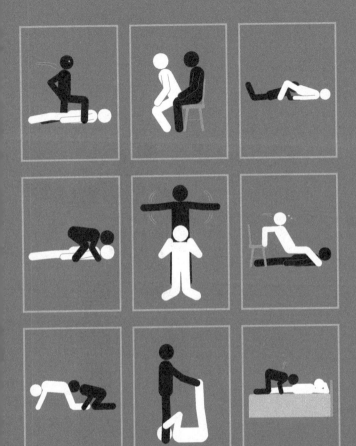

Beginner's Sexercises

Sexercise can be HARD WORK, and whether you're "like a virgin" or more of a "sex bomb", it's always a good idea to ease into things. These simple sexercises will get your love engines purring nicely, while leaving you wanting more. Get it on and sweat it out, guys and gals— it's time to pump it up (figuratively— we're not promoting penis enlargers here, although each to their own).

The How-Low-Can-You-Go Lunge

DIFFICULTY RATING: BURN RATING:

With your partner lying flat on the floor, stand at their feet with your weight evenly distributed—get a good look at their naked form while you do this. Perform lunges, alternating between legs, dropping forward and down over their body. Get as low as you can, grazing their nether regions or tickling their nipples as you descend. Take it in turns to be the lunger and lungee.

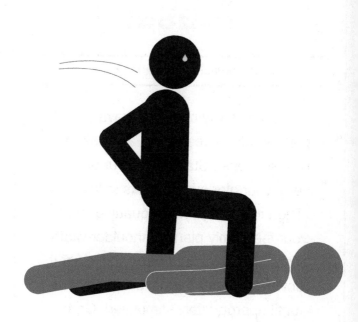

The Squat Teaser

DIFFICULTY RATING: 🍆🍆 BURN RATING: 🔥🔥🔥

Grab a sturdy chair and have your
partner take a seat—nice and naked is
probably best. Stand with your back to
them, your glorious buttocks in full view.
Then it's time to start squatting. With
your feet firmly planted shoulder-width
apart, push your butt back and lower it
down onto your partner's lap. Repeat
until appropriately stimulated. Or, to
make it a little harder, try not to let your
parts touch theirs, and hold the squat
for as long as you can both bear it.

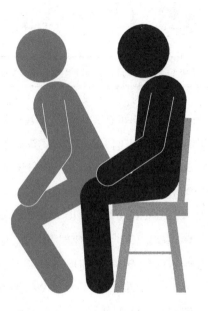

The Bridge of Thighs

DIFFICULTY RATING: 🌶🌶 **BURN RATING:** 🔥🔥🔥

Lie on your back with your
knees pointing towards the sky
(or a mirrored ceiling if you're so
inclined), feet set far apart. Squeeze
your buttocks tight and raise your
hips off the floor or bed into a glute
bridge while your partner goes down
on you. As soon as you lower your
butt back down, trade places. This
works your glutes and core, and
keeps their mouth in shape too.

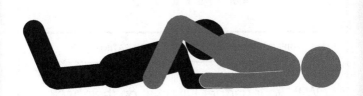

The Wet-Weather Mountain Climber

DIFFICULTY RATING: 🍆🍆🍆 **BURN RATING:** 🔥🔥

With your partner lying flat on their back, crawl up over the top of their body, only resting on your hands and feet. You will look like a robotic gecko, so offset this unsexy hilarity by licking all parts of them as you go. When you get to the top of the mountain (that's their face) roll over and have them do the same to you in return.

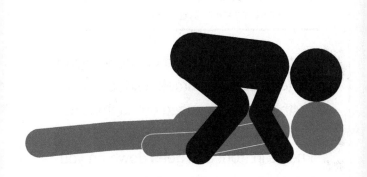

The Circular Sensation

Get your limbs geared up for whatever
(or whoever) comes next. Stand
with your arms raised out to the side
at shoulder height as your partner
kneels in front and goes down on you.
Keeping your arms raised, rotate them
in a circular motion, forwards for a few
seconds, then backwards for a few
seconds, without letting them drop.
Your shoulders will start to scream,
but probably not before you do.

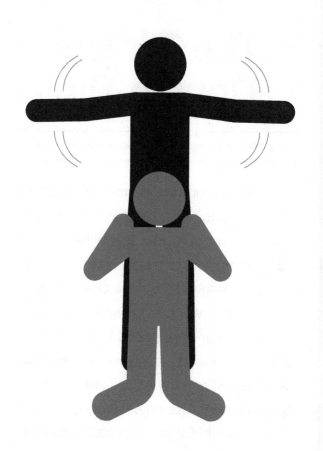

The Triceps Double-Dip

DIFFICULTY RATING: 🌰🌰🌰 BURN RATING: 🔥🔥🔥🔥

With the penetrating partner lying flat on the floor, position a chair over their legs. Facing them, with your feet either side of their shoulders and your hands resting on the edge of the chair seat, lower yourself down onto their erect penis, strap-on or dildo (lubed to the max). Using your triceps, push yourself back up and repeat as long as you can stand it. Bend your legs for an easier ride or keep them straight for an extra-hard workout.

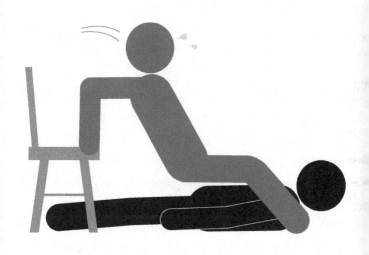

The Hamstring Hey Diddle Diddle

DIFFICULTY RATING: 🍆🍆🍆🍆 BURN RATING: 🔥🔥🔥

Here's a great little sex move that's got legs! Kneel down together with the rimming receiver in front. The person behind holds on to their partner's ankles and leans forward to tongue-tickle their lover's fancy (and provide a useful counterbalance). As they do so, the partner up front should lean over toward the floor, tightening their hamstrings as they go and putting their arms out to catch themselves. Then they push back up and repeat (or not, if they're particularly enjoying what's going on to the rear).

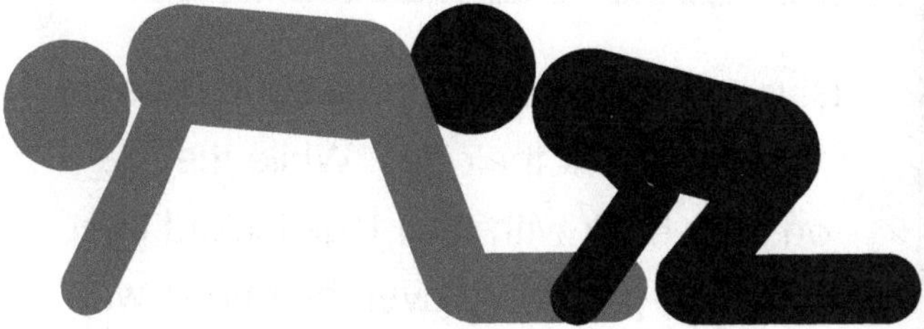

The Ab-racadabra

DIFFICULTY RATING: 🍆🍆🍆 BURN RATING: 🔥🔥🔥🔥

Give your lover a little peekaboo session
as they work their abs. While they lie
on their back with their legs locked tight
together, you stand over their head with
your arms extended out in front of you.
Your supine sexpot grabs your ankles
and raises their legs up without bending
them to meet your hands. If they can
reach up for a little handjob in between
reps, all the better. Core-blimey!

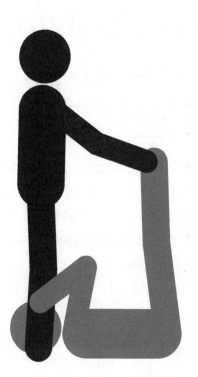

The Bowing Blowy

When it comes to giving head, there's no room for being half-hearted. But there is room for half press-ups. Position yourself over your partner's reclined lower half on your hands and knees. With your arms shoulder-width apart, lower yourself up and down. Take the time when you're down there to whip up a little treat with your tongue. Your shoulders will thank you, and so will your partner.

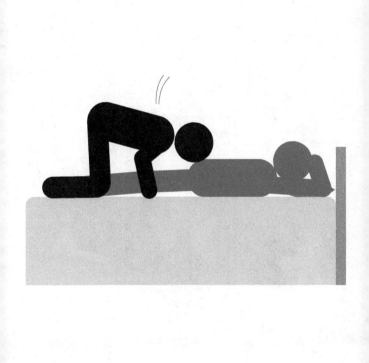

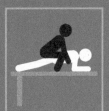
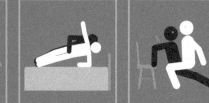
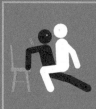
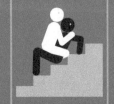
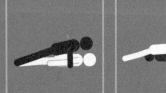
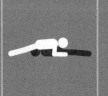

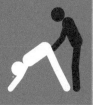

Advanced Sexercises

No one likes to blow their own horn
(that's what your partner's for!), but
if you've not felt the burn yet, things
are about to go up a bedpost notch.
In this section you'll find ball-busting,
love-muscle-aching sexercises to
transform your bedroom routine
for the sweatier. Keep your mind
focused and your buttocks clenched
as you power through to the climax.
Now you're really gonna get it!

The Plank Poker

DIFFICULTY RATING: 🍆🍆🍆🍆 BURN RATING: 🔥🔥🔥🔥

Find a flat surface raised a little higher off the ground—the dining table should do. Lie on your stomach, resting on your forearms and then, with your toes curled under, raise up in a classic plank position. Prepare for penetration! While you hold the pose, your partner enters you from behind (a penis, dildo or finger will do here). If penetration ain't your thing they can get all gropey however you like.

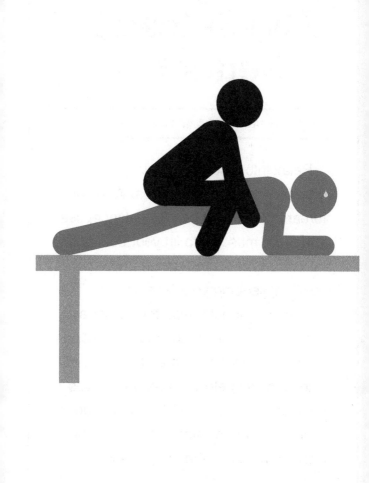

The Sideways Seduction

DIFFICULTY RATING: 🌶🌶🌶🌶 **BURN RATING:** 🔥🔥🔥🔥

Relax into a suitably sexy spooning position, lying on your sides. With your forearm flat on the bed for balance, use your core muscles to lift your bodies off the bed as far as you can in a side plank position, keeping your legs straight. The little spoon should raise their other arm up for balance, while the big spoon does a sneaky reacharound and gets things going down below. Lower yourselves back down to the bed—big spoon, don't stop that manual stimulation—and then back up again as the temperature rises.

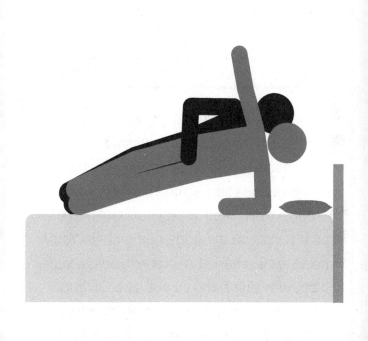

The Squat Tester

DIFFICULTY RATING: 🌶🌶🌶🌶🌶 BURN RATING: 🔥🔥🔥🔥🔥

If you've mastered The Squat Teaser (see page 34) then you're halfway to nailing this bad boy. Get a chair and assume a tricep-dip position—with your legs straight out in front, resting on your heels, and your hands on the edge of the chair. You'll need to be wearing a strap-on or just your birthday suit if you've got a penis. Your partner straddles you, facing the chair, primed for penetration or locomotion.

As you perform dips, your partner assumes a squat position to meet you, cheering you on as you feel the burn.

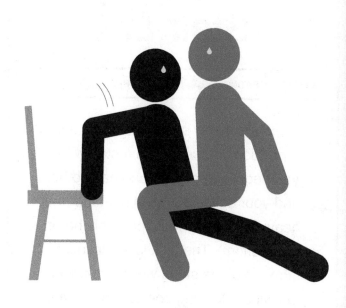

The Sexy Stair Lift

DIFFICULTY RATING: 🍆🍆🍆🍆🍆 **BURN RATING:** 🔥🔥🔥🔥🔥

Find a suitably sturdy staircase and position yourselves on a step with your legs wrapped around each other and your uglies bumping big-time (the heavier person should probably be on the bottom). The trick is to make it to the top of the stairs while remaining entwined. Moving one step at a time, with your biceps bulging and your pelvis engaged, hoist yourselves up to the top.

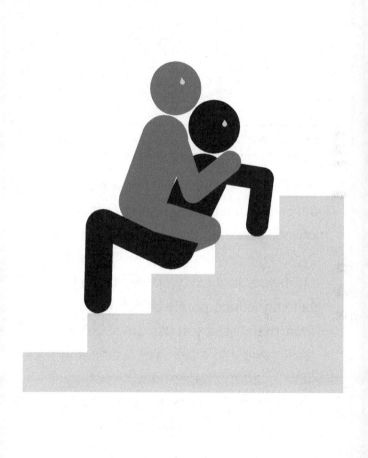

The Big Mission

Press their buttons while your master your push-up technique with this muscle-motivating take on missionary. You'll need your legs positioned hip-width apart, with your feet firmly planted if you're planning to incorporate penetration. See how many reps you can get in before collapsing into a big sexy cuddle. For those lacking upper-body brawn, try The Bowing Blowy on page 48 instead and build up to this shoulder-shredder.

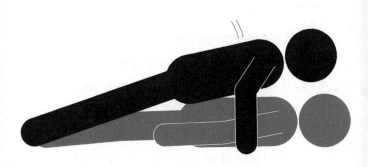

The Stacked Sixty-Nine

DIFFICULTY RATING: 🍆🍆🍆🍆 **BURN RATING:** 🔥🔥🔥

Get better acquainted with each other's
nuts and bolts by reclining top to tail,
and then get to work with your yaps,
nibbling, sucking and licking to your
heart's content. If that's starting to
sound a bit too easy, you'd be right.
Once the ecstasy is setting in, take it
in turns to perform a plank over your
partner's body while still continuing on
your oral odyssey. Try to fight temptation
to give in to the pleasure. Tap out
when you need to take a breather.

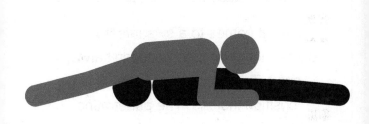

The Leap Froggy

DIFFICULTY RATING: 🍆🍆🍆🍆 **BURN RATING:** 🔥🔥🔥🔥

When it comes to a sweat-fest worth carb-loading for, doggy doesn't always cut it. Try this amorous amphibian position instead. The penetrating partner kneels while their froggy friend positions themselves in front, resting on the soles of their feet instead of their knees and placing their palms on the ground for support. This classic crouch offers penetrating pleasure and a mighty fine thigh and glute workout to boot.

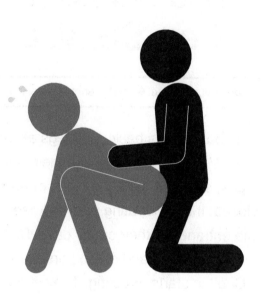

The Scissor-Leg Samba

DIFFICULTY RATING: 🍆🍆🍆🍆 BURN RATING: 🔥🔥

One partner lies back, their legs akimbo in a V shape. As they work their inner thighs, slowly fanning their legs open and closed, the penetrating partner kneels at the entrance to their candy cave. Ready to get up close and oh-so personal? El Capitan starts thrusting. They should squeeze their buttocks too for some sneaky glute-toning as they thrust.

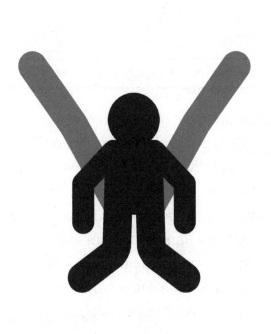

The Marble Arch

DIFFICULTY RATING: 🌶️🌶️🌶️🌶️🌶️ BURN RATING: 🔥🔥🔥🔥

Gear up to get guns as strong as stone. The penetrating partner sits on the bed with their legs straight, while their partner sits on top facing them and gets acquainted with the Little General (or Lady Penelope . . . or whatever euphemistic nickname you desire). Both your arms should reach back between each other's legs for support. Time to hammer it hard, but pace yourself. You're going to need triceps of granite to make it all the way to climax.

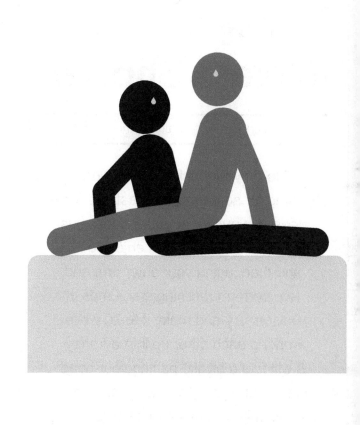

The Mutual Meteor Shower

DIFFICULTY RATING: 🍆🍆 **BURN RATING:** 🔥🔥🔥

Lie on your backs side by side.
It's time for some mutual masturbation—
pleasure yourself or your partner (just
make sure you're both enjoying it),
and then, using your outer arm and
leg, perform reclining star jumps in
unison. Try and make it to 20 while
working each other up into a frenzy.
It will feel a bit like patting your head
and rubbing your stomach at the same
time, only with much more pleasure.

The Downward Doggy Style

DIFFICULTY RATING: 🍆🍆🍆🍆 **BURN RATING:** 🔥🔥🔥

Bending at the waist, one partner descends into a downward dog pose (for those non-yogis, this means your body should be in an A position)—pressing through their heels and the palms of their hands, with their butt pointing up towards the sky. While they breathe deeply, their partner can begin to pleasure them from behind.

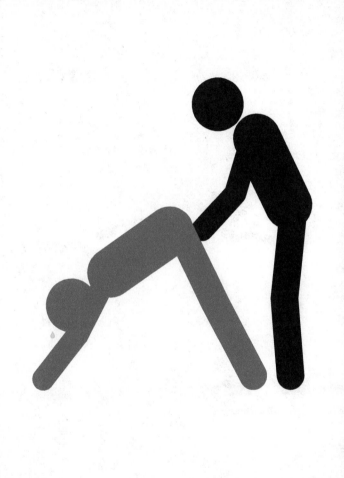

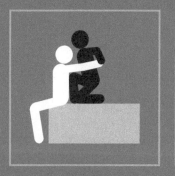

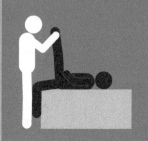

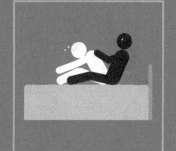

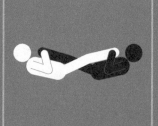

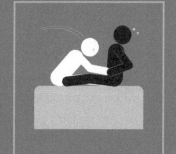

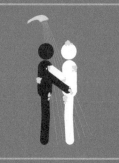

Cool Down

Oh. My. God. Your toes might be curling
and your nerve endings are probably
freaking out, but we're not quite done
yet. All that hard work will go to waste
if you don't take care of your body and
cool down after you come. So take a
quick breather, and then regroup for
this final frisson of post-coital bliss.

The Impressive Chest

DIFFICULTY RATING: 🍆 BURN RATING: 🔥

Open up that upper body (and show off your assets) with this simple chest stretch. The stretching partner sits on the edge of the bed, legs together and arms wide open. The supporting partner kneels behind, one knee (or third leg) positioned against their partner's back. Starting at their armpits, the supporting partner runs their fingers out towards their partner's hands and slowly pulls their arms backwards, stretching on the chest. If your partner's got a cracking pair or a svelte set of pecs, you can enjoy them all the more from this angle.

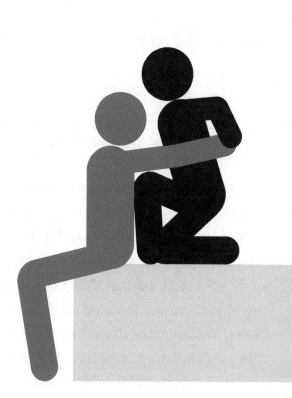

The Ham-String 'Em Along

DIFFICULTY RATING: 🐾🐾 BURN RATING: 🔥🔥

Time to tease your partner into submission for another forage around the forbidden fruit. Lie on your back with your arms by your sides and your legs out straight. Your partner then takes each leg in turn, raising them up towards the ceiling to stretch out those hammies. As they do so, start to pleasure yourself. You'll be glad you're all limbered up because you'll soon be back in the sack.

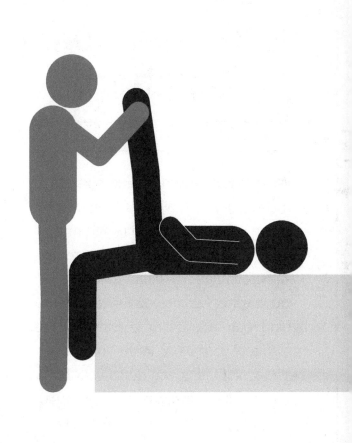

The Remote Reacher

DIFFICULTY RATING: 🦶🦶 BURN RATING: 🔥🔥

Want to wind down with an episode
of your favorite reality TV trash-fest?
Flat on your backs and miles from the
remote? Never fear. Sit facing the remote
with your legs hip-width apart. With
your partner easing you forward from
behind (ooh-er!), putting pressure on the
middle of your back, lower your head
between your legs and reach your arms
forward. Alternatively, one of you could
just get up and grab the damn thing.

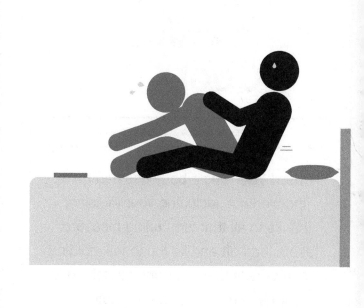

The Toe-Curling Cool-Off

DIFFICULTY RATING: 🍐 **BURN RATING:** 🔥

Phew! Your whole body has had quite
the workout, including your tootsies,
thanks to all that toe-curling pleasure.
Take a load off and lie top to tail, holding
each other's feet. Flex and stretch your
partner's paws out, as you both try
not to squirm with ticklish glee. A little
massage oil should work a treat too.

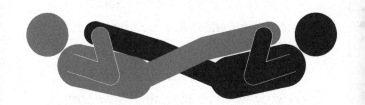

The Thigh's
The Limit

DIFFICULTY RATING: 👣👣 **BURN RATING:** 🔥🔥

Sweaty and satisfied, sit facing
each other with your legs open and
outstretched as wide as possible. Hold
hands and stare lovingly into each
other's eyes. Intense, right? Now comes
the stretching part. Take it in turns to
pull each other forward. When you're
being pulled, bring your upper body
forward and downward—within licking
distance of your partner's inner thighs.
Hold for 10 seconds, then pull further
if you can and hold for another 10.

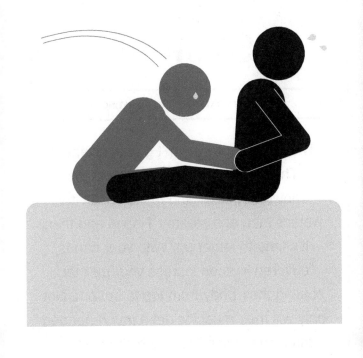

The Shower Shimmy

 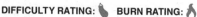

Thought things couldn't get any wetter? Think again. Make your way to the shower together and make out till the water's nice and steamy. Hop in and then it's time to lather up. With your hands covered in suds, caress your partner, coating their body from top to bottom. Not only will their muscles get a much-needed massage, you'll be stretching yours as well as you soap them into sensual bliss.

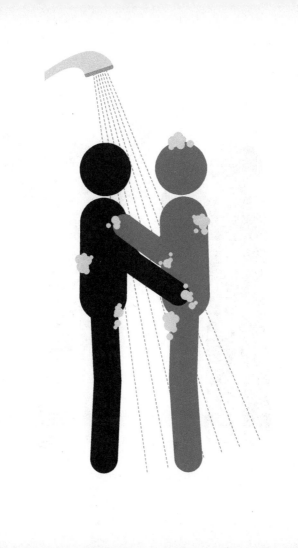

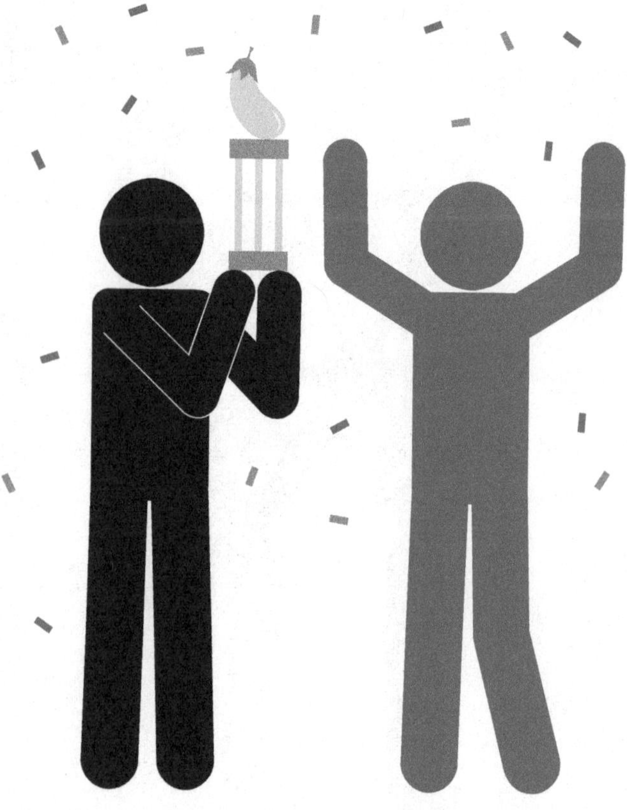

Congratulations

After much huffing and puffing, to-ing and fro-ing, thrusting and sucking, you've finally made it to the end of this glorious sexathon. Well done you! And while there are no podiums on which to stand (the end of the bed should work just fine) and the national anthem isn't going to play (you can always ask your partner to hum along), you should consider yourself a gold medal winner in the Humping Olympiad.

Log Your Workouts

Date	Description	Score out of 10

Date	Description	Score out of 10

Checklist

☐ The Dry Hump

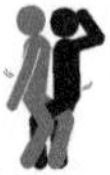

☐ The Strip Teaser

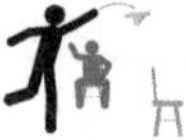

☐ The Locked-Lips Limber

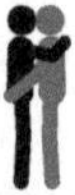

☐ The Squat It Like It's Hot

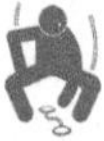

☐ The Throwdown

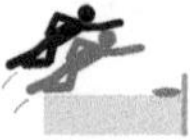

☐ The Big Switch

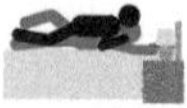

☐ The Lubricator

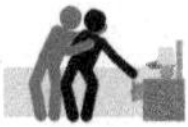

☐ The Safe-Sex Salsa

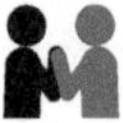

☐ The Condom-nundrum

☐ The How-Low-Can-You-Go Lunge

☐ The Squat Teaser

☐ The Bridge of Thighs

☐ The Wet-Weather Mountain Climber

☐ The Circular Sensation

☐ The Triceps Double-Dip

☐ The Hamstring Hey Diddle Diddle

☐ The Ab-racadabra	
☐ The Bowing Blowy	
☐ The Plank Poker	
☐ The Sideways Seduction	
☐ The Squat Tester	
☐ The Sexy Stair Lift	
☐ The Big Mission	
☐ The Stacked Sixty-Nine	
☐ The Leap Froggy	
☐ The Scissor-Leg Samba	

☐ The Marble Arch

☐ The Mutual Meteor Shower

☐ The Downward Doggy Style

☐ The Impressive Chest

☐ The Ham-String 'Em Along

☐ The Remote Reacher

☐ The Toe-Curling Cool-Off

☐ The Thigh's The Limit

☐ The Shower Shimmy